YOGA

Meditation, Mindfulness, and Weight Loss.

Yoga Guide to Healthy Living.

Johnny Fitness

Disclaimer Notice:

Table of Contents

Introduction

In this fast-paced world, it is very easy to be overwhelmed and stressed. I mean, there are always deadlines to beat, to-do lists to follow, studies to pursue, you have to catch up with friends, you need to look for ways of earning money and you still have to somehow maintain your sanity in the midst of all these. Many of us may cave into the pressure and basically shut down and this is where problems begin. Your stress levels increase, you seem always anxious and fearful, you never get enough rest because the anxiety and the stress can make it impossible to sleep, and you never seem to enjoy life. If nothing is done to address the situation, the pressure would be too much for your body and the next thing is that you have high blood pressure, diabetes, heart diseases and other health conditions because of the anxiety and stress. I am sure this is not what you want your life to be. So, what are your options?

Have you tried meditating? By simply spending five minutes to meditate daily, you bring some form of sanity, as the meditation quiets and calms your mind. Meditation helps you to get a moment of calmness that helps you deal with the daily challenges. This book will look closely at yoga and meditation, and their importance in the modern world.

It's not just about stress. The book shows you how yoga can help you with your weight loss and also with the way that you view the world, helping you to find peace within that inner self that you rarely come into contact with. The world's busy pace stops you from doing that. More and more people are finding that integrating yoga meditation into their lives means addressing some of the problems that life inflicts upon the unwary.

As you get more and more experienced with yoga, you find that you are more able to meditate. It's not easy at first, but with this guide, you have all that you need to make the most of the experience and use it to help you to make your life a much more peaceful place in which to reside. Once you do, you will wonder why it took you so long to actually take responsibility for your own happiness because through yoga that's exactly what you are doing and this book shows you how.

Meditation and Yoga

Despite all its popularity, very few people today can actually be able to define what meditation is. Some perceive it as concentrating on something mentally, while others deem it as imagining something that provides peace and satisfaction. All these definitions have one purpose: to slow down, and completely stop the ceaseless activity of our minds. These definitions do not explain meditation clearly but rather help you to understand what meditation entails, since it is technically very hard to stop your mind altogether.

The truth is meditation is a mental state of thoughtless awareness. It is a state of awareness, and not an act of doing. Either you are in this state or you are not, regardless of what you are doing in life. In fact, you can be in meditation while you are going on with your daily activity, while another person can be in something else apart from meditation while sitting in a lotus position on the top of a mountain. When you consider the various definitions of meditation, you will find that meditation is often defined as taking a moment to ponder or sit quietly. But true meditation is much more than this.

Meditation is actually a three-step process that results in a state of consciousness that brings bliss, clarity, and serenity. Our normal state of mind is in fact, quite abnormal. When you receive sensory stimuli, you tend to react in a completely uncontrolled way, while telling yourself you have great control. You bounce from one thought to the next and follow with your physical and emotional reactions. At different times, the same thought can lead to diametrically opposite reactions. For instance, you may see a dog and then start a thought process that reminds you about a pet dog you once had and loved. Another time, emotionally, you may see the same dog and fear it may attack you, and start having paranoid thoughts, get uptight and fearful physically.

The second phase illustrates concentration. It is actually the first step in meditation, and is the beginning of gaining control over your mind, and ultimately, your life. The process is very simple, and may seem very easy to do, but it involves a few tasks more difficult to master. Ideally, what you need to do is pick a subject or object to place your focus on, and then concentrate exclusively on it without diversion. If you decided to concentrate on love, for instance, you would start by relaxing your body, sit in a comfortable posture; quiet your emotions, and then start repeating the term "love" over and over again. The problem is that throughout your life, your mind has been your master and it won't relinquish this position easily. It will divert your attention in a bid to trick you back into compliant slavery, usually by providing you with a tantalizing distraction. When this happens, you need to see yourself being distracted, and then get back to concentrating on the subject of your meditation.

The third phase illustrates meditation. Here, you are in a state of unbroken attention. The difference between meditation and concentration is given in the classic example of pouring oil into a bowl from a bottle. The oil starts by dripping out a drop at a time, and this is concentration. The oil then comes out in a steady stream, and this depicts meditation. If you really take a closer look at the process, you will see that when the oil was coming out in drops, it caused a splash with each drop, and the droplets of the splashing can be compared to the distractions that interrupt your concentration. But when the stream becomes steady, it starts flowing effortlessly. In the same way, when concentration metamorphoses into meditation, concentration becomes deeper and deeper spontaneously and effortlessly.

Meditation is a part of yoga. In fact, yoga and meditation are totally and exclusively interrelated. By definition, yoga is a traditional way of life encompassing practice and thought aimed at wellbeing and good health; emotional, mental and physical – that is said to end in nirvana or moksha (emancipation or liberation). That said meditation is an elaborate part of yoga, it being one of eight limbs. The others are: Yamas (Restraints or don'ts), Niyamas (Observances or do's), Asanas (Poses and exercises), Pranayamas (breathing techniques and exercises), Pratyahara (Regulation of the senses), Dharana (Concentration), and Samadhi (super conscious state).

How Does Yoga Work?

Yoga uses pranayam or breathing techniques, focused concentration of specific parts of the body, as well as asanas or postures to incorporate the body with the mind, and the mind with the soul.

Before you get to try out yoga, you need to practice or limber up a little and one of the best methods I know to get accustomed to the meditation side of yoga is to lie in a quiet room and try to think of absolutely nothing. You will find it impossible to sustain this lack of brain activity, but that should be enough to convince you that yoga is the right choice for you because your mind needs rest. Now, lie down on a bed and support your head with a pillow. This is merely an exercise in relaxation that is helpful before you start yoga. Close your eyes and focus on your toes.

Now tense your toes and then relax them. Feel the tenseness to its extremes, feel the relaxation to its extremes too because both are important to your focus. Focus on each part of your body in turn, firstly tensing the part in question and then relaxing it. When you have finished, make sure that you get up slowly and that you take a few moments to go back into the busy world. Your mind needs that relaxation and once you begin yoga, you will get all the help that you need. Why not just do relaxation sessions? Because it's not complete and it's not enough to help you to begin to tune your mind and body as yoga will. Yoga is more complete as explained below.

The body

Yoga asanas (poses or postures) are helpful in conditioning your body. Yoga poses are thousands in number, and in Sanskrit, they are referred to as kriyas or actions, mudras or seals, and bandhas or locks. A kriya concentrates on the effort you need to move energy up and down your spine. On the other hand, yoga mudra is a movement or gesture to concentrate awareness or hold energy, while a bandha involves the technique of regulating muscular contractions to focus awareness. These are all helpful to the body. You will find that as you go through the process of the different exercises in a correct manner, you will benefit from them, in that your body will become supple and you will be able to hone in on areas that are problematic and thus help your weight control.

The mind

Yoga teaches you to concentrate on specific parts of your body in order to focus on your mind. This awareness keeps your mind and body connection sharp, and does not allow plenty of time for external chatter. The focus is instead internal, between your body and your head. This is healthy from the point of view that your mind gets a rest and that also helps you to build up mental energy to take on the tasks of the day more efficiently.

The spirit

Yoga utilizes controlled breathing in order to integrate the mind, body, and spirit. These breathing techniques are known as pranayamas. When disintegrated, prana means life force or energy, while yama refers to social ethics. The controlled breathing of pranayamas is believed to regulate the energy flowing in your body. The spirit is the important part in yoga because it helps you to feel some kind of realization spiritually which is not dependent upon any specific type of belief. With a little understanding of yoga, let us now look at the benefits of meditation and yoga.

Benefits of Yoga and Meditation

The many possible health benefits of yoga and meditation, including reduced risk of diabetes and improved cognitive function are well documented. Studies have even suggested that meditation and yoga can influence gene expression, perhaps even minimizing the expression of genes linked with inflammation. Recent research has also revealed that lifestyle changes, including less stress, moderate exercise, and improved diet could actually reverse the aging process at a cellular level. That's powerful stuff and worth bearing in mind especially if you feel that you do have inherited illnesses within your family, as the yoga exercise can help to stem that illness and make you much stronger.

When practiced together, yoga and meditation strengthen the mind and body connection, thus improving your overall wellbeing and fitness. Several styles of yoga merge meditation with the physical routines that use controlled breathing during the yoga poses. You can actually meditate without even practicing yoga by just relaxing, clearing your mind and focusing on controlled breathing. When used consistently, both yoga and meditation have proven benefits. You will also feel very energized and that's important as well because it means that you are able to take on more difficult and time consuming tasks with ease because your brain is sharper.

Stress management

Practicing yoga on a regular basis can help reduce stress responses in your body. When you reduce the inflammatory response to your body's stressors, you will reduce your risk of stress related conditions like cardiovascular disease and high blood pressure. Meditation is similarly an effective stress reducer used to help reduce panic disorders, anxiety, and agoraphobia (an anxiety disorder). Thus, when you learn the meditation process, you are able to be more in control of your life and can stop stress and anxiety in their tracks. This helps you long term because stress can kill. It can cause physical illnesses to manifest and your control of those illnesses will be much more likely.

Improve Flexibility

In the current society, we are plagued with sedentary jobs that require workers to sit for the most part of the day. This results in reduced flexibility, fitness, and muscle mass. Furthermore, office work enhances neck and shoulder strain because of hunching over the computer all day. Yoga poses concentrate on lengthening and stretching the muscles. Increased flexibility will go a long way towards helping you with daily movements like bending and lifting, as well as in improving sports performance. In fact, several athletes integrate yoga into their workout routines to improve and maintain flexibility. It also helps you to concentrate on posture and this is extremely helpful for those who are working in sedentary jobs and is likely to contribute to firming up flab and making the body much more trim and neat.

Emotional boost

Yoga and meditation both provide a general feeling of wellbeing and improve mental focus. Most yoga disciplines revolve around an upbeat theme. For instance, the philosophy of anusara yoga looks for the good in all things, and is designed for an uplifting experience centered on the celebration of the heart. Meditation delivers an emotional boost through deep relaxation, and you can do it anywhere. You can take a ten-minute meditation break right where you are to give yourself an emotional boost. Simply close your eyes, concentrate on relaxing your muscles, and start deep breathing.

The emotional side of yoga is one of its strong points because it makes you feel inner strength and that helps you to get back to basics and remember who you are and get back into synch with body and mind so that you can cope better with the stresses and strains of life.

Better diet

Practicing yoga can improve your body awareness and fitness, and ultimately lead to better eating habits. In turn, this leads to increased self-esteem and the motivation to take care of your body. Practicing yoga or meditation is a behavior modification skill that can help you improve your general wellbeing. Yoga instructors will suggest that you drink more water and this helps considerably with keeping the body hydrated. Most yoga practitioners find that good balanced food goes with the lifestyle and are encouraged to eat foods that are very healthy.

Improved health

Getting more exercise, eating healthier and reducing your stress levels can only result to better health. Life today is stressful due to the long working hours, stressful situations, and little sleep, anxiety disorders, allergies, and a long list of stress related complications. Incorporating meditation or yoga in your life can improve the quality your life. When you have improved health, it means that you can be able to participate in more physical activities, and feel better in the things you do every day. Let us now look at some meditation techniques that you can practice today for stress relief and happiness.

Johnny Fitness

Meditation and Meditation Techniques

With the hectic demands and pace of modern life, more and more people are feeling stressed and overworked. It always seems like there is just not enough time to get everything done. Our tiredness and stress makes us frustrated, impatient and unhappy. It even affects our health. People are often so busy that they feel there is no time to stop and meditate. Actually, meditation gives you more time by calming your mind, and making it more focused. A simple 10 or 15 minute breathing meditation can help you overcome your stress, and find some balance and inner peace. It can also help you understand your own mind. You can learn how to transform your mind from negative to positive, from unhappy to happy, and from disturbed to peaceful.

Imagine if, while you were reading, an antelope walked up to you. You would probably stop reading and thinking about whatever it is that is on your mind, and focus entirely on the antelope. Or even more realistically: imagine driving home from work, thinking about what you are going to eat for dinner, when you are pulled over by a police car. Even if you are obeying the law, your attention may now switch to the speedometer and rearview, as recollections of the workday disappear as you silently urge the police car to change course. While you may not want an antelope or a police car following you, it is helpful to take on that focused attention these experiences beg. Meditation is exactly the process of doing that – cutting through your mind's static and finding focus. Meditation offers both a range of health benefits, including stress management, helping with depression, heart disease, and high blood pressure, and is as well something you can tailor into your daily lifestyle. If you want to try it, you don't need to take a visit to a monastery or a doctor's office. Meditation is not a mystical thing, but is basically your trained attention. As a beginner trying out meditation, you can do the below three simple meditation techniques just about anywhere, anytime. Before you start, the best advice would be to go slow, and be gentle and compassionate with yourself. Chances are your mind will wander while trying to focus, so don't be overly stressed when it does.

Walking Meditation for Stress Relief

This simple, traditional practice is well suited for stressed out people in modern society. It will also be very useful for people who work in office environments and will help them to be able to concentrate in a more focused way when they have heavy duties such as conference calls and need to hone their minds ready for questions or for public speaking.

Find a suitable space outside and walk at a medium or slow pace, while focusing on your feet. Try to become aware of when your toes touch the ground, when your toe is raised back upward, and when your foot is flat on the ground. Feel as your foot rolls on the ground. Keep in touch with your sensory details: a pull of the sock here, a tingle there.

In case your mind wanders, which it most definitely will, bring your attention gently back to your feet. By doing this, you are developing a skill of being aware when your attention wanders into default mode, and getting back into focus. This can go a long way towards helping you become more present and in control of your attention on a daily basis, especially when stressed out.

Walking Meditation can be described as a mild form of exercise. Start by designating a specific place and time to practice, and when you become comfortable with it, try it while walking to the office, home, or just about anywhere.

Novel Experiences (Meditation for Happiness)

Remember how you shift into focus mode when you unexpectedly meet an antelope or when you see a police car. You tend to escape your brain's jumble of daily thoughts when you experience something out of the ordinary. In the same way, you may pay more attention to a loved one when you meet him/her after a month, as opposed to when you see him or her every day.

Try this:

-When you get home at the end of the day and meet your family, pretend like it's the first time you have seen them in thirty days. You may be faking this feeling, to an extent, but it may be useful to think about transience; there are only a limited number of evenings you will have with these people you adore. For instance, if you have an eight-year-old daughter, she will be off to college sooner than you know it then she will be done with college, move out of the house and get married.

-Another way you can support this feeling is to aim for acceptance. The human brain is a fault-searching machine. Your first goal for the first ten minutes at home should be to try to improve nobody.

This practice is not restricted to family. Try to create a fresh view of just about anyone you come across every day, including neighbors and co-workers, to get you into focus mode. The newness of the situation that you are creating means that you are more aware of things that you would otherwise not notice. It helps you to see things from a new light and that's always healthy and also means that you appreciate the things which surround you in your day to day life much more than you usually would.

Gratitude Exercises

What do you think about when you first wake up? Perhaps: What am I going to wear? Where is my coffee? When is my first meeting? Even while you are still yawning and stumbling out of your bed, you probably often dive into default mode headfirst.

As a general rule of thumb, try to delay that for two minutes. Use the first two minutes of your day after waking up to find focus.

-Close your eyes and imagine you are waking up this morning, picturing the layout of your bedroom.

-Next, think about the first person that you are grateful for, and bring their face in front of your eyes. People tend to cry when they try out this exercise but that's a good sign because it's letting your emotions wake up to the world as well.

The best time to practice this technique is in the morning, as well as when you are stopped at red lights, while waiting in the checkout line, or between appointments. When you start practicing this exercise, you will stop feeling as if you are missing out on life, and start to see all the good things around your life that you have been gifted with. You will also find that you are much more aware of people and positive toward them, and that the positivity that you aim at other people will come back a thousand times more and make you very happy to be alive.

Positivity has the effect of a magnet. It will mean that you are in touch with more positive people and that they will enjoy your company, making your life more rewarding and very positive in your interactions with others. That always helps you to feel good about life.

Yoga and Yoga Techniques

It turns out that everything you have ever loved has a pattern. Every experience of feeling swept away; every extraordinary, and divine moment, followed a similar experiential melody. The main reason why most people struggle to find happiness in their lives is that they failed to realize when they were totally happy and absorbed. They fail to recognize they were actually acting in a certain, repeatable way.

Imagine you are in a yoga class. It all starts with some breathing. The whole goal is to relax and leave your stress behind. Once you settle yourself in the present moment, you start to do poses, sometimes vigorously such as in Bikram, other times deliberate such as kundalini. While different classes vary, depending on the school, the purpose remains the same: yoga's objective is to unify all the parts of yourself while breathing, and then flow with the movement of all the positions. Each session ends in meditation and breathing. The aim is to feel the change in your spirit and body. When you first start, you were likely entangled in the chaos of reactive living. You were carrying on with what you were supposed to do, and at the pace of expectations and demands of others. However, at the end of a session, you feel stable and at peace with yourself and the world.

The reason why yoga works is because it follows the pattern of every focused human experience. The best moments usually happen when your mind or body is stretched to its limits in a conscious effort to achieve something hard and worthwhile. But what most people have not learned is what to do to create these moments of satisfaction. The best moments of your life, your sweet spot, follow a simple pattern. They start when you center yourself. However, you have to be present before you can stretch to your limits and decide what you want to do that is hard and worthwhile.

The first thing you need to do is decide to slow down and be where you are. This is what takes place when an athlete does their routine or ritual before a game. It is what musicians do when warming up their instrument or voice. It is the writer lighting a candle before writing words on a page, or a chef sharpening his knives. You can't simply jump into a moment of happiness and total peace. You first need to activate the part of your brain that is responsible for happiness. The second thing you need to do is to focus, or ponder on what is most important to you. Your sweet spot is achievable because your frontal lobes, the part of your brain that focuses on thinking, fires on all cylinders. If it wasn't, you would be needy or wanting, anxious or nervous. When you decide to experience or think about what you are doing at the moment giving it your full attention that is when the cravings and nerves quiet down. Yoga is simply focusing your mind wholly on your breath, or what your body is feeling as you move through a pose. Giving a talk is possible when you concentrate on telling the listener to look at things differently, or on telling a great story, rather than worrying about whether the audience will like you. A parent should be responsible when he/she wakes up in the middle of the night to soothe a child. They are fatigued, and may not even know what is wrong. However, the voluntary decision to comfort the child is what brings fulfillment and absorption.

The final step to finding your sweet spot is what yoga is so effective in, and most people never realize is essential. You need to self-reflect how you are feeling in order for an experience to be registered as valuable. For you to store the memories of a peak experience in your brain, to realize an experience is worth repeating, you have to consciously distinguish what has just happened from the moments in your life where you are reacting to what a situation demands or what others want.

This is what takes place when you meditate at the end of a yoga session, or when you stretch after a run. It is when you sit with a professional or coach to assess a recent event, or when you write in your journal to register how you really feel after a date. Your sweet spot is all about what you feel when you feel at your best and when you are focused. Those are the experiences you want to recur every day. The moments you want more in your life are patterned with a formula. Self-check, focus and center: These three behaviors are at the center of why yoga is effective, and the 3 phases of any experience you have loved.

So, next time you feel alone, grumpy and angry, keep in mind that you already have areas of your life where you have found your sweet spot. Simply maximize on the next super sweet experience that you have by finding the pattern and re-using that pattern over and over in your life, so that it becomes a living joy. Another experience that helps you to find your joy is greeting the sun in the morning and yoga has the perfect pose for this. It is a series of exercises which are called the sun salutation and it stretches all of your muscles and then relaxes them, making you feel more energized and about to carry out your day in a very positive manner.

You will learn all of these different poses later, but for the time being, remember that there are moments that are joyful within your life. You may not yet have registered those moments or the lead up to them, but when you find the repetitive nature of joy, you are able to tap into it whenever you need it in your life and that's a valuable resource. Let us now move to some yoga poses and the warm up necessary before you start yoga.

Body Warm-up Exercises Before Yoga Exercises

It is not natural to take your body from having no exercise at all to being immersed in yoga exercise. Yoga exercise is very good for you, but it's important to warm up before you start feeling the benefit of the exercises that an instructor will give you or that you choose to do on your own.

Warming up

Stand with your legs slightly apart and with your feet flat on the floor. Hold one arm out in front of you and shake it. It may sound strange but this shaking effect allows your muscles to loosen up ready for the exercises. Shake the wrist, shake up to the elbow, and circle your arm so that your shoulder gets a little exercise. Then place the arm back by your side. Repeat these warming up exercises with the other arm. Then hold one leg out in front of you in a naturally comfortable position and shake it. Shake your ankle, shake up to your knee and then shake the whole leg. Relax and place the foot back into its original place on the floor. Repeat the process with your other leg.

Move your head to the right, keeping the rest of your body straight, slowly bring it back to center and then move it to the left. Repeat this several times as this helps your neck to lose some of the stiffness and stresses that life places upon it.

Shoulder rolls

These are very helpful for mobility. Stand with your feet slightly apart and raise your arms outward in front of you, locking the fingers of one hand to the fingers of the other. Keeping your fingers locked, take your arms over your head in a rolling motion or circular motion coming back to the same position at the front of your body. Repeat this warm up exercise five times in one direction and then five times in the other direction.

Sun Salutation for beginners

From a standing position, move your hands as if you were about to say a prayer. Then inhale and reach your arms out as far as you can to the sides and then up to the sky. As you exhale, move your arms to the side and just like an elegant swan, bend your body forward. Hold onto the bottom of your legs and look forward and feel your body stretch.

There are many versions of the sun salutation, so do not be confused. This version is simply for beginners who have never done yoga before and does not encompass some of the more complex movements that more advanced students would do.

Now that you have done your swan dive and have your arms against your legs, inhale and bring your arms back out to your sides as you stand as tall as you can. Then lift the arms up as high as you can reach with your fingertips pointing up toward the sky to greet the sun. Hold this position and breathe in and then exhale as you bring your arms out to the sides down to your body and then back into the prayer position.

Repeat this several times. It's a great warm up for first thing in the morning or to do on the beach when you have been lazy and want to get into a serious yoga practice but haven't prepared yourself in any way. It makes you feel very satisfied and happy and it also makes your body feel ready for the yoga session ahead.

Why preparation is important

Preparation is important because you can't go from a tense, nervous body directly into expecting your body to respond in a positive way to all the stretches that yoga imposes. Thus, you need to work when you are a fair distance from meals, avoid heavy meals, eat healthy food and keep your body hydrated at all times by drinking sufficient water. All of this helps to prepare you for yoga and will set you in good stead for your first sessions of regular yoga exercise. With this kind of preparation, your yoga exercises will not seem like hard work at all and will simply be a continuance of your yoga routine.

Yoga Poses for Weight Loss

As you start on the yoga poses, ensure you have a yoga mat as it helps provide some padding to avoid the hard ground. Ensure that you practice the poses outlined below at least three times a week, holding each pose one time for three to five deep breaths, unless otherwise stated. For each exercise begin with the main move. If it is too hard, do the easier variation. On the other hand, if it is not challenging enough, try the harder option. For quicker results, hold every pose for five to eight breaths, and increase the repetitions by two or three.

Main pose: Crescent (Firm thighs, hips and abs)

Stand with your feet together, arms at sides and toes forward. Breathe in and raise your arms overhead, reaching your finger-tips towards the ceiling. Breathe out, and bend forward from your hips, bring the hands to the floor. Breathe in, and as you breathe out, step back into a lunge (right leg lengthened and on ball of foot; left knee bent around 90 degrees, knee over ankle). Breathe in and raise your arms overhead and gaze forward. Hold, get back to standing, and repeat while stepping your left leg back.

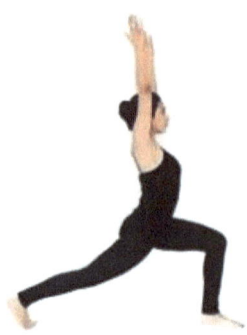

Make it harder: From the end position, breathe in and arch your torso, head and arms backward, and gaze at your fingertips. This makes it harder because the arching of the torso and the looking up at your fingertips works your spine and your neck and will eventually lead to increased mobility. However, if this is too hard, do not force yourself to take the hard path, since you can injure yourself if you try to take on these exercises too quickly.

Make it easier: lower your right knee until it touches the floor as you step back into a lunge, and rest your hands on your left thigh. This makes the stretching a little easier for those who have impaired mobility or who have not exercised for a long time. Be very careful never to push your limits too far.

Main move: willow

Stand with your arms at sides and feet together. Place the sole of your left foot inside your right thigh, with your knee bent to side.

Touch your palms in front of your chest for two breaths. On the third inhale, extend your arms up, with the fingertips pointing the ceiling. Breathe out, and while inhaling, bend your torso to the left. Breathe in and straighten. Repeat for three to five times, while pressing your foot into thigh, and then switch sides.

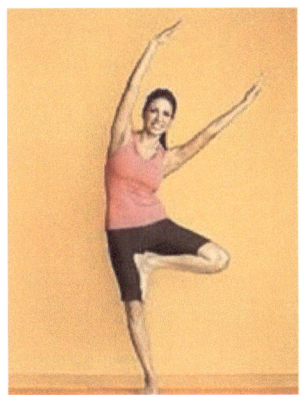

Make it easier: Place your left foot on calf, or point your toes to the floor for balance. Take it slowly and try to find a position that is comfortable and where you can still retain balance. This may be harder for older students who may want to start by holding onto a chair with their right hand until they have established the right balance. Never take risks if you suffer from vertigo or any ear problem that gives you balance difficulties.

Make it harder: Close your eyes as you bend and balance. Closing your eyes places all of your focus on what you are doing, rather than being able to use focal points to help your balance.

Your inner self gives you those focal points and although it sounds easy to just close your eyes, it's much harder to begin with. As you gain in inner peace through the practice of yoga meditation, however, you will find this easier to handle.

*Main move: Hover

Start in a push up position while on toes with your arms straight, body in line from your head to heels, and your hands below your shoulders. While exhaling, lower your chest towards the floor, bending your elbows back, abs tight and arms close to your body. Maintain a few inches above the floor.

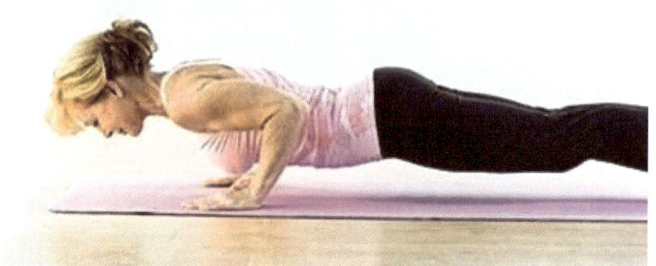

Make it easier: Start on your knees and hands, and walk with your hands forward until your body is in line from your head to the knees. Remember to stop when the exercise becomes too hard. It isn't about pushing yourself but it is about finding your own personal limits.

Make it harder: As you hold the hover, lift your left leg six to twelve inches, hold, and then lower. Do three to five times, and then switch your legs. This will help your calf muscles and your muscles around your lower back to firm up.

Main move: rocking boat

Sit with your knees bent, hands on thighs, and your feet on floor. With your torso straight, and your head in line with your body, lean back approximately 45 degrees, raising your feet so that the toes are pointed and the calves are parallel to the floor. Breathe out, and as you breathe in, lower your legs and torso three to four inches so that the body forms a wider V shape. Breathe out and raise your legs and torso. Repeat three to five times. The amount of times that you repeat depends upon how comfortable you feel with the exercise. Don't ever push your exercises too quickly.

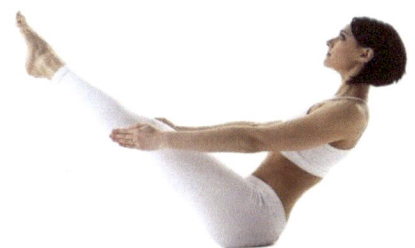

Make it easier: Hold the back of your thighs with your hands, and your legs bent. Lower your torso only. If you find this hard, work into the exercise gradually. Yoga is not supposed to hurt. It is supposed to make your muscles stronger and your body more toned but it should not be thought of as a punishment, more a relaxation and being at one with your body.

Make it harder: Once you get to the wider V pose, extend your arms above your head. This takes a little bit of practice but you can achieve it when you are confident at forming the V position and raising your hands above your head will reinforce the strengthening of the stomach area and abs.

These exercises are very good for your body but when doing them, remember that you need to use your mind to concentrate on your body position. Body and mind must always work together. Regular practice of yoga exercises will make you feel fitter, will help to tone the body and will also mean that you feel better in yourself. Interspersed with yoga meditation sessions, you can exercise between three and five times a week, depending upon how much time you can set aside for your yoga practice and upon whether you feel that meditation or exercise is what benefits you the most. Thus, if meditation serves you well and your body doesn't need too much exercise, then meditation more frequently will be a positive thing.

Yoga For Happiness

Find a yoga mat, a bolster, or any other firm pillow, two blankets, two blocks and a strap. Props can give you support so that your body can move into a comfortable stretch, instead of too much strain in a pose or too much stretch.

When using props to support the torso, ensure that the height of your prop is comfortable for your back. Rather than a bolster, use a folded blanket if less height under your back is better for you. It's a very individual thing and you have to find the balance that works best for your body and your comfort levels.

Maintain active poses for twenty to thirty seconds each, and repeat them twice to each side. You can stay in resting and supported poses for as long as you are comfortable. These help you to shape up and tone your body or the parts of the body which are aimed at by a particular exercise. You will know which parts these are because you will feel it within you and can use the exercises that tone up the parts you need to trim more frequently than other exercises, but do try to balance your exercises to keep your whole body supple.

Breathe fully and deeply in all poses, with even exhales and inhales. If you feel pain in a certain pose, now is the time to come out. You won't gain by pushing your body through pain.

In the supported positions, you can close and cover your eyes using an eye bag. On the other hand, if you are comfortable with your eyes open, you can leave them to soften and shift your gaze inwards towards the back of your head instead of reaching outwards. Gaze within, as opposed to without.

Let us look at a simple pose that you can do when feeling sad and low and you would feel much better afterwards.

Easy reclining pose

Lie down with your head supported slightly above on a folded blanket, and your spine supported on a bolster. With your knees bent out to the sides, allow your legs to relax by crossing your ankles. Use blankets to support your knees and thighs in order to release tension in your legs. Let your arms rest by the side of your body. Switch the cross of your ankles after a few minutes. Open your chest further by holding your elbows and then placing your arms overhead.

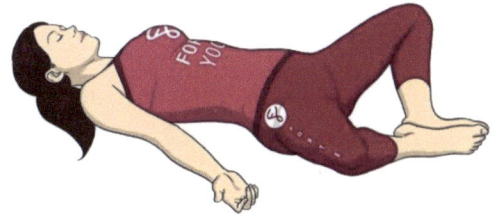

In this relaxed pose, become aware of the flow of breath throughout your body, especially in your chest and abdomen. Acknowledge the connection between your emotions and your breath.

Your breath tends to be short and caught when you are feeling tense or anxious; and if you are feeling depressed and empty, your breath may be uneven and shallow. Try to balance between your inhalation and exhalation, and identify how your feelings are affected. Your feelings can become softer and smoother along your breath. Experience the knot at your diaphragm/navel area rising to give you a sense of self-worth and personal power.

These exercises should help you to feel revitalized and are wonderful exercises for your wellbeing. Do practice them because they will help you considerably to feel that the yoga is working and is giving you a great sense of happiness.

Read on to the next chapter because in the next chapter, we want to show you how you can use yoga meditation to make you feel wonderfully energized and ready to take on the world. This can be done in the quiet of your own home or you can use the outside spaces to give you inspiration to draw from. Many people meditate in areas that are naturally beautiful because it inspires them and gives them positive energy, which is then used through the process of meditation to make the mind and body come together in harmony.

Yoga Meditation and How It Can Help You

Although we have covered other areas of yoga meditation, we haven't gone into detail about when you can use it and how it will help you. Meditation, which is taught in yoga, is to make your mind aware of the moment in which you are. Many say that mindfulness meditation is a good way to go and combine this with yoga meditation although I would personally stick to one system or another. The problem with mixing the types of meditation is that some types concentrate on the feelings within the body, while others concentrate on external forces and they are a little contradictory. To learn the discipline of yoga meditation, you look inward and find a harmony within your own body. This is very important because it helps you to feel happy about who you are and to understand all the messages that your body is trying to tell you better than under other circumstances.

It is worth remembering that you can do this at any time and that if you are feeling the stresses of life, this may be your body's way of telling you to slow down and meditate. Carry your music with you if you want to use this in a public place or when you are out and an MP3 player or something of this nature is ideal.

The kind of music that you need for this immersion into meditation is Tibetan Chakra meditation music. You can either buy yourself a CD or find YouTube Videos that can be converted into MP3 and which are very useful for the purpose of meditation. While you meditate, you look inward, so close your eyes because this is important to meditation. The idea is to cut out external interruptions, except the music. The music isn't for listening to. It's for bathing in while you concentrate all of your thoughts on your breathing.

The ideal position to do this kind of meditation is to take the lotus position and to place your hands so that your middle finger touches your thumb, and place these onto your knees. However, this isn't obligatory. Many people think that it is, but it can make you feel inhibited when you are in a public area. Thus, as long as the pose that you take is totally comfortable, then you can actually meditate without anyone being aware of your actions and without being conscious that people are watching you. This is particularly relevant to new yoga practitioners because the lotus position is hard at first and you should never try the full lotus where your feet are tucked in without guidance. It is far better that you find a comfortable sitting position where your back is straight at all times for this type of meditation. Having a straight back means that your body is able to keep its posture and the messages that run from one area of the body to another are easily aligned.

Close your eyes, turn on your music and let it embrace you. Don't listen particularly, because the idea of this type of music is immersion. Concentrate on your breathing. As you breathe in, feel the air filling your lungs and hold it for a moment. Then, breathe out and as you do so, be conscious that you breathe out a little longer than the inward breath and that the breath comes from the abdomen area of the body.

If you find that you can do this better without the music, that's fine too. Concentrate on the counting of the breath entering your body, the held breath and then the breathing out and the movement of the upper abdomen area of the body.

You can practice this for up to half an hour or even longer if you are in a situation where you have time on your hands and want to enjoy basking in the relaxation that this form of meditation gives you. When you have finished your meditation process, come back into the world gradually. Don't startle your senses. In other words, gradually turn down the volume of the music, gradually open your eyes, keeping your breathing at the same pace. Never get up abruptly as it takes a little time for your body to come back to that full consciousness that is needed for every-day life. Enjoy your meditation and enjoy the energizing that it gives to your mind and your body. If you are working in a busy environment, this can be every bit as healthy as a visit to the gym at lunchtime and if you can find a park where the area is not too filled with noise and distraction but where you can get close to nature, this is a good way of giving yourself extra energy for the afternoon that lies ahead. Similarly when you are travel-ing, if you stop to meditate, gradually come back to your normal breathing and opening your eyes, you will be able to start your traveling again feeling refreshed and ready for it, rather than being overly tired.

Yoga For Stress Relief

Let us look at some poses for stress relief. These are particularly good because they hone in on different areas of the body and help you to feel less strained and stressed by the world around you. Practice these whenever you feel that you can add them to your day because they really will help to get rid of stress and make you feel happy in your life. Remember, when doing exercises, do not push yourself. Yoga isn't about punishment or suffering. It's about release.

Down dog

Breathe in and then step back to downward dog while holding for a minute. Allow energy to flow through your arms and through your sit bones. Draw your shoulders away from your ears and keep your neck long. As you exhale, press down through the heels in order to help stretch your Achilles tendons, calves, and hamstrings. Point your right leg up and back, and then open up your hip.

To shift from the down dog to a low lunge with the hip open, rise up on the ball of your left foot, then bring your right knee towards your chest. Lift your butt up high and point the toe of your left foot while placing your right foot next to your right hand. With your fingertips under your shoulders, breathe in to a flat back. Position your left knee down on the mat. Bringing your torso back over the pelvis and with your hands on the front knee, hold the stretch. Reach back using your left hand and catch your left foot for more sensation, stretching the heel towards the left glut.

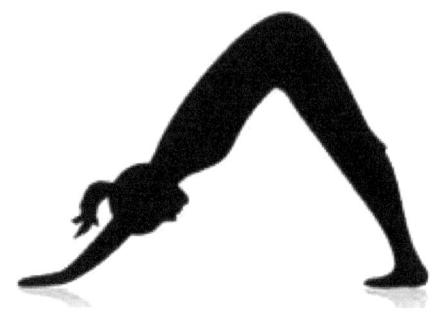

Pigeon pose

Place both of your hands under your shoulders on the mat, coming onto your fingertips. Heel-toeing your right foot towards the left wrist, place your left leg back to achieve a better stretch. If you find your hip off the floor, fill the gap by holding a block or towel. Fold your upper body over your shin as you breathe out, and then lower down onto your forearms. Unfold your toes.

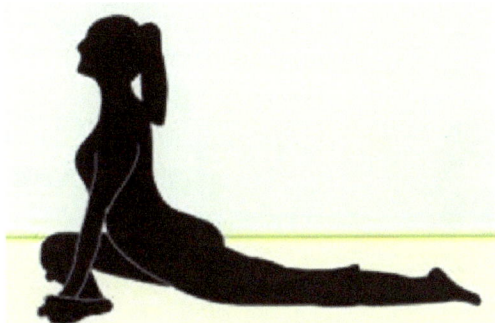

Half bound ankle pose

Place your right hand over your head and bend to the left to grab your left calf using your right hand. Bring your forehead to the outside of your left knee as close as you can. Take a couple of breaths, breathe in fully, and sit up while exhaling.

Seated forward bend

Stat by sitting on your yoga mat then bend towards the center, flex both of your feet, and hold them that way. With your right shoulder opened up, extend up your arm while you exhale. Your fingertips should point towards your opposite toes. Breathe in, stretch your spine, and hold deeper while exhaling. Breathe in once more, and come to a seated position as you breathe out.

Johnny Fitness

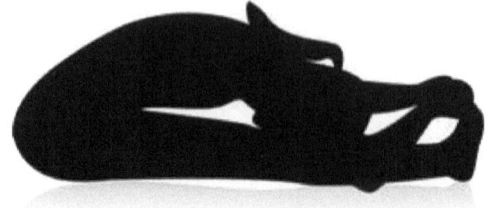

Yoga as a Life Choice

You may not know it at this stage, but talk to experienced yoga practitioners and what they will all tell you is how yoga helps them to center their lives. It helps them to relax. It helps them to keep all the body muscles in trim and it helps to keep the ligaments in good order. It helps them in other ways too. When you become more conscious of your body's needs, you make a life choice. It's unlikely that you would follow a yoga practice with a binge of overeating, because yoga teaches you to respect your body and to listen to its needs. Thus, you will find that yoga gives you a new perspective which helps you to become fitter and much more responsible about your body. You will know which foods, for example, are the best foods to feed yourself because your comfort and discomfort levels are affected by what you eat.

The thing with yoga is that it places the responsibility for your wellbeing into your hands and gives you control of how energized you are. Thus, overeating and overindulgence in unhealthy practices won't be an issue because if you are listening to your body and are honed into its needs, you won't be looking for substitutes for happiness. People who are depressed often overeat all the wrong things as a way of compensating themselves. Binge eaters do it, but when you have yoga on your side, you balance those emotional feelings and don't have the same need and can still reduce depression, stress and discomfort levels all on your own.

You also get to learn all of your weaknesses and learn that the way forward is to work on those weaknesses to eliminate them. Yoga is very positive and it's a positive reinforcement of your own importance. People with self-esteem issues learn how vital they are to the order of things and learn to find that center of self-love that stops them from being self-destructive.

Thus, as you can see, yoga becomes a way of life. Does that mean you will be eating lettuce leaves for the rest of your days? Not really. It does mean that you will have a great sense of taste and will know all of the different foods that make you feel good inside and that may surprise you. Lettuce leaves may not do that for you, but there are so many foods that are a positive influence that you may find you experiment more with your foods and avoid those foods you know to make you sluggish and unhappy.

Yoga practice will help you sleep better. If you are one of those people who says that they don't need sleep, then you are fooling yourself. The human body was made in such a way that the hours of sleep are used by the different elements within the body for a time of repair. If you do not sleep properly, your body doesn't have that time to repair itself and eventually you will become a victim of lack of sleep. Sleep is also necessary for the release of the subconscious thoughts that everyone needs. Imagine your subconscious as a little child inside you that needs playtime. If you deprive the body of sleep, the subconscious may as well become a child, trapped inside, who is not permitted movement.

During the different levels of sleep, your subconscious needs to work and may produce dreams, but may just be working on sorting out all of the thoughts of the day and putting them into some kind of order. Let your body sleep correctly and you will feel better and will be able to perform your yoga exercises in a much more productive manner.

From the moment of reaching adulthood, you have a responsibility to your body and to your mind. Yoga, as part of a balanced lifestyle, helps you to fulfill your responsibilities to self in such a way that your body and mind will thank you for it. You will know when you need water. You will know when you need a change of environment, and you will be able to give your body all of the support that it needs to feel healthy and strong. Look at the ways in which yoga meditation can be introduced into your life and you not only have a strong body, but you have a mind that is honed to the body and that is able to give you comfort, happiness and satisfaction that you are on the right track.

When you take up yoga, you are taking up a lifestyle. It's not just an exercise routine. It's a way of life that helps to sustain your mental attitude and your physical abilities.

Conclusion

If you want to maintain your sanity in this fast-paced world, you need to learn spending a few minutes meditating and even practicing yoga each day and incorporate it into your life. I hope this book has provided you with all the information you need to start practicing yoga and meditation for stress relief, happiness and weight loss. The next thing you need to do is to start practicing what you have learnt and experience a difference in your life.

The difference that you will feel when you start to see yoga as a viable alternative to other lifestyles is that you will see that it's a complete care system. It doesn't just help your fitness levels. It helps your mental understanding as well and brings you very close to being at one with the world that you live in as well as having mind and body working in harmony.

There is a whole world out there waiting for you and when you start to practice yoga on a regular basis, you may find that you want to do this alone, or you may find that at first, you need the support of others within a class situation. This is a good choice if you are unsure of the positions and want to know if you are handling them correctly. You will also get moral support from other students, which is always a good thing to consider when you are starting something that you have never experienced before.

Invest in a good mat, have a towel with you to use as a pillow and wear clothing as advised by your instructor and very soon, you will find that yoga isn't something new. It has lasted for centuries because of its benefits to mankind and once you are comfortable with your yoga practice, you too will be benefiting from that age old way of life that anyone can make a part of their lives, in order to reap the numerous benefits available to those who take yoga seriously. You will be very glad that you did and you will find that you can maximize the potential of your body and mind and feel wonderful about the effects of meditation and yoga exercises if done on a regular basis. I know that when I started, I found it hard to accept the theories behind yoga. Now I am enthused beyond words as I walk into my 20th year of practice and have embraced yoga as a way of life. You too can do this and find out for yourself that there's a whole new world out there, waiting to embrace you, your body and your mind and help it to develop its full potential.